Written By:
Bryan Miles, Medical College of Wisconsin
Edited By:
Drew Porter, University of Wisconsin School of Medicine and Public Health
German Larrain

Table of Contents

Introduction

Getting accepted into medical school is hard. Really hard. In 2017, 51,680 applicants sent out 816,153 applications to medical schools around the country. Well over half of these applicants faced rejection, not getting accepted into even one school. But don't get discouraged, this won't be you! I have used my knowledge and insight gained from reviewing hundreds upon hundreds of essays to create a simple, interactive, and all-inclusive guide that will ultimately help you perfect one of the most crucial elements of your application. An element that is not just a number, but an intimate representation of why you'll be an amazing doctor and why admissions officers should not hesitate to accept you into their medical school…

Of course, I'm talking about the personal statement! I remember being in your position applying to medical; feeling completely overwhelmed by the task of trying to convince admissions committee members why they should pick me over thousands of other qualified candidates, in merely 5,300 characters. I sought out many resources, but they all lacked the essential details that make up truly memorable personal statements, so I decided to change all that and guide you through this often-frustrating process!

I have had the privilege of helping countless applicants create unique and memorable personal statement essays. This workbook is designed to help you avoid common pitfalls that may hurt your chances of being accepted and focus on key elements that will ultimately set you up for success.

How is this book set-up?

First, I'll answer all of the frequently asked questions of the personal statement, so you fully understand all the specific ins-and-outs of this important essay. After you understand this foundation, I'll walk you through 5 interactive steps that will help you create your own effective personal statement! Then, I'll go over some final dos-and-don'ts before having you grade your own essay using Bryan's Black Bag's rubric. Towards the end of the book, I'll walk you through two personal statement essay examples, specifically what they did right and what they could improve upon. Finally, I'll finish by taking you through multiple drafts of a third personal statement example, and outline what it ultimately takes to turn a good essay into a great one.

Well, enough chit-chat. You bought this book to learn how to write a personal statement, so let's get after it!

Frequently Asked Questions

How long should the personal statement be?

You are allotted 5,300 characters--which comes to about a page and a half of text single-spaced. More important than the length, though, is whether you prove what is in your thesis. Obviously, you do not want it to be too short, so I would aim for at least a page minimum. Beyond that, it really comes down to whether you drew the reader in, presented your argument, and, most importantly, convinced them thoroughly of that argument. What I've seen is that most find themselves struggling to cut characters out, not add them.

When should I start writing my personal statement?

We recommend beginning the process of writing your personal statement several months ahead of the due date (which is the first day you are able to submit your centralized application). This changes from year to year, but generally falls in early June. Given the rolling nature of medical school admissions, there is absolutely no reason not to be submitting on the first day, or at least very shortly thereafter. Those several months beforehand do not need to be spent toiling away for countless hours a day. The idea is that, if you give yourself several months, then you can work through the process slowly and methodically. With the help of this book, you will know *where* and *how* to begin!

Unfortunately, you will more than likely write several, "fine-tuning" drafts once the appropriate and compelling content is in place. Taking time to start this essay and receive feedback earlier sure beats stressing-out in the weeks before the deadline, forcing you to deliver a subpar product.

When should I have a rough draft done by?

If we quantify the several months alluded to above as 3-4 months, then I would say you want a respectable rough draft two months prior to the submission date. This will vary from person to person, depending on your schedules and ability to power through the fine-tuning process, without sacrificing quality of course! Being more specific, a respectable draft means you have worked through this book in full and have reflected on and written each element of the personal statement, including the introductory and closing paragraphs, and the body paragraphs. In short, the content you wish to use in support of your thesis must be in place. These two months are reserved for largely grammatical changes by you and others. Who you should entrust to provide feedback on your personal statement will be touched on in a moment.

When should I have a final draft completed?

This has been touched upon, but I will clearly state it once more. Your final draft should be done in time to enable you to submit your application on the first possible day, or very, very soon thereafter. This stems from the rolling nature of medical school admission.

Do admissions committee members even care about my personal statement?

ABSOLUTELY! Many schools have cut-offs for the objective metrics of the application, like your MCAT score and GPA. Once you reach those, you have shown your academic prowess and capabilities, so they move-on and want to see who you truly are as an applicant. This is where the extracurricular and personal statement essays come-in. To some extent, many pre-meds have the same extracurricular experiences, so the personal statement is something that can really differentiate you. It is a blank slate for you to talk about why this is your purpose in life, and why you will make an exceptional physician. The admissions committee members are looking at thousands upon thousands of applications, but your essay can set you apart from other candidates, many who also have excellent objective metrics. This is not intended to stress you out, but rather to emphasize the importance of the personal statement.

Who should I have edit my personal statement?

There are two types of edits: those grammatical in nature, which touch on punctuation and syntax, and those that zero in on content. In the case of the personal statement, that content is going to revolve around how well your body paragraphs support your thesis statement. The grammar edit can be done by anyone with a proficient English background. These are not the types of edits that will truly transform your personal statement though. It is your choice of content and the delivery of supporting stories (don't worry, there is much more on this to follow!) that really elevates a personal statement to something truly special. Therefore, the pool of people who can provide critical content insight is much more limited. An obvious starting point is other premeds, but you ideally want someone who has successfully matriculated, as that shows they understand what is necessary to create a strong personal statement. Some schools have pre-med advisers, but unfortunately not all are cut from the same cloth. I was truly blessed to have an incredible pre-med adviser who continually provided invaluable insight and feedback. This is not the case at all institutions and you will be left to determine for yourself whether your adviser can provide what you need. Last, there are reputable companies out there than can turn your personal statement from an average submission into one that is truly magnificent. I have a track record of doing just that and would love to continue to help you with this process – If interested, email me at bryanmiles17@gmail.com to learn about my review packages and use the code "**workbook10**" to receive an exclusive 10% discount off any package!

How much overlap do I want between my extracurricular activity essays and my personal statement?

This is a tough question to answer. Your extracurricular activity essays, (especially your three most significant ones) like your personals statement, represent you in a subjective manner (versus objective metrics like your MCAT score and GPA). If you've already written these essays, you probably have fully stated what you believe are your stellar traits, and recited the stories and/or insights that actually back-up your claims. However, our recommendation is to temporarily push all of this out of your mind as you initially construct your thesis. The thesis of your personal statement does not center on your extracurriculars per se, as it is a reflection on why you wish to pursue medicine and why you are perfectly suited to thrive in the career. There can be some overlap in the anecdotes and/or insights you choose to support the points in your thesis. By some, I would suggest sticking to only a single, overlapping element because you want to try and cast as diverse a picture of yourself as possible.

Step 1 – Write Your Thesis

What is a thesis? To put it bluntly, it is the core argument for your entire paper. This is a creative essay in a sense, but the organization you learned for writing persuasive essays is crucial (if you happen to have forgotten, this all begins with your thesis). That being said, the thesis of any effective medical school personal statement needs to answer two important questions:

1. Why do you want to be a physician?

2. Why are you going to be an amazing physician?

This is what you are setting out to prove. If you fail to clearly answer these questions, the entire piece will lack direction and efficacy, but most importantly, your argument will not be clear to the reader. This will make them lose focus on the supporting evidence for your argument and could ultimately hurt you as an applicant.

With this in mind, here are some "good" reasons to be interested in medicine, answering the "Why do you want to be a physician?" question. Note, they may appear simplistic here, but can always be spruced up in an actual thesis:

- To help people.

- Being drawn to the challenges presented by medicine.

- The ability to continue learning and improving.

- The rapidly evolving landscape of medicine.

- The unique teamwork and comradery.

- Being fascinated by the human body and medical technology.

- Some combination of the above.

Here are some "bad" reasons to pursue medicine:

- The money (this actually is a fallacy given the steep opportunity cost--sorry but true).

- The prestige.

- Being the boss.

Here are some "good" qualities to highlight in yourself as an applicant, essentially answering the "Why you will be an amazing physician?" question:

- Compassion and empathy
- A strong work ethic
- Perseverance
- Adaptability to adversity
- Natural curiosity
- Communication skills
- Ability to function within a team
- Leadership skills

For the sake of completeness, here are "bad" qualities to avoid mentioning. Most applicants would never blatantly state any of these, but you want to avoid even the possibility of what you are saying being construed as meaning one of the following:

- Egotistical
- Not punctual
- A deficiency in any of the above "good" qualities

Now let's build your thesis!

1a) Why do you want to be a physician? Make your own bulleted list below.

_____

_____

_____

_____

_____

_____

_____

_____

_____

1b) Now turn this into a coherent sentence (I want to be a physician because...).

_____

_____

_____

2a) Why will you be a great physician? Make another bulleted list below.

_____

_____

_____

_____

_____

_____

_____

_____

2b) Turn it into another coherent sentence (I will be an excellent physician because…).

_____

_____

_____

_____

3) Lastly, combine 1b and 2b into one coherent sentence. And voila, you now have your thesis statement.

_____

_____

_____

_____

Thesis Statement Checklist:

□ Thesis statement answers "why you are interested in medicine" question.

□ Thesis statement answers "why you are going to be an amazing physician" question.

□ Thesis statement is clear and coherent.

Up Next: Let's build upon this thesis and create some truly epic body paragraphs...

Step 2 – Write Your Body Paragraphs

Believe it or not, the hardest part is over! You are no longer a captain-less ship or a pilot-less plane. You now have direction, governed by your awesome thesis statement. Although many might try to hammer out an introductory paragraph after writing their thesis, your next step should be creating effective body paragraphs. This will ensure that your body paragraphs stay focused on your thesis and more than likely make your introductory paragraph easier to write (outlined in the next step). Each body paragraph has a specific theme—again, as set forth by the thesis statement. The simplest and most effective recipe to follow is to devote the first paragraph to discussing why you are interested in the field of medicine, while using the subsequent three paragraphs to highlight the respective traits that are going to make you an excellent physician.

> Body 1: Why are you interested in medicine?
> Body 2: Awesome Trait #1
> Body 3: Awesome Trait #2
> Body 4: Awesome Trait #3

Going back to the "Why medicine?" element of your thesis statement, we now need to expound upon that in the first body paragraph. The most effective way to convince the reader of your passion is with a story. We refer to this as showing, rather than telling. By drawing them in with a story, you convince them, beyond a shadow of a doubt, of your love for medicine. If you merely say "I am interested in medicine because of X, Y, or Z," your argument is much less compelling. Additionally, your story is much more powerful if you play an active role in it. By this, I mean YOU are the star of the show, the lead character; everything centers around YOU. This is as opposed to a passive example, where you are merely an observer, watching someone else be great. You are the applicant! You are the one you need to build up!

A perfect example of something passive is shadowing. Shadowing, by its very definition, is passive. You are a shadow, not the owner of the shadow. We want the latter, not the former. Last, zeroing in on particular details of the story pays dividends. For instance, say you worked at a summer camp where you made huge contributions to the program. If you detail this, sure, it is both a story and an active example, but speaking in generalities will not move the reader as much. Instead, you want to focus on a particular kid with whom you had a unique relationship and influenced in a positive way. This is where the money is! To quickly summarize:

- Show, don't tell.

- Be active, not passive.

- Be as detailed and focused as possible--painting a clear picture that brings emotion into the story.

In the spirit of "show, don't tell," here is me showing you an example rather than just telling you what to do:

Read the following narrative and think about what is lacking within it…

During my freshman year, I became a volunteer in the Emergency Department. While volunteering, I was able to observe the hospital staff. This opportunity helped solidify that I have chosen the ideal healthcare profession for myself. I also obtained my Nursing Assistant Certification and started working at a Senior Living Center. I was unaware of the immense positive impact this experience would have on my life. I love seeing smiles on my residents' faces and showing them someone cares—especially when their families do not visit them regularly.

First and foremost, the author is not showing the reader anything. Instead, they are merely telling them about two activities they took part in, much like reciting their resume. Boring! Additionally, nothing about this paragraph is active. This is a by-product of their lack of storytelling and results in the reader being left unconvinced of their passion for medicine. Moreover, details are sparse. Details help the reader be convinced of whatever it is you are attempting to prove — passion for medicine in this case. So, how would you improve upon this paragraph? Here is where I'd start:

During my freshmen year, I began volunteering in the Emergency Department. One particular encounter stands out. Emilie was a little girl who unfortunately stepped on glass shards at a local beach. She came in sobbing hysterically and bleeding somewhat profusely from her foot. While the physician took stock of her injuries, I cozied up to her side and inquired about her stuffed animal, a rabbit. His name fittingly was Thumper. I asked when she got him and about the things they loved to do together. As she detailed their adventures together, including watching Frozen and running through the back yard, her tears slowed, and she forgot all about her foot. This truly magical ability to care for people in their time of need captivated me. Hungry for more, I began working at a nursing home as a certified nursing assistant. Gladus suffered from dementia and sadly her family had stopped visiting several months prior. Eager to fill the void, I paid special attention to her care plan, embellishing it with her favorite treat each week, home-baked chocolate chip cookies. Although she struggled to voice her appreciation, her smile told me all I needed to know. Ultimately, experiences like this reinforce my career path.

In contrast to the previous paragraph, this one incorporates everything we recommend. First, the author's passion for medicine is palpable from the two stories shared: one from the emergency department and another from the nursing home. Second, the stories focus on the author, highlighting their aptitude for the field, rather than unnecessarily showcasing someone else. Last, the abundant details give you a chance to really sink your teeth into the narrative. Ultimately, I think it is obvious which paragraph is stronger and better convinces you of the author's desire to pursue medicine.

Now it's your turn! Let's use what we just talked about to start working on your body paragraphs…

Body #1: Brainstorm stories, in accordance with the above bullet points, that demonstrate your deep-seated passion for medicine:

_____

_____

_____

_____

_____

_____

Body #1: Now, pick the most powerful ones and turn it into a succinct body paragraph:

_____

_____

_____

_____

_____

_____

_____

_____

_____

_____

_____

The next three body paragraphs are organized according to the three traits mentioned in your thesis supporting the claim that you will be a kick-ass physician. The order of the body paragraphs follows the order of their appearance in the thesis.

Body #2: Brainstorm stories to support your first trait. Again, show, don't tell; be active, not passive, and zero in as much as possible:

_____

_____

_____

_____

_____

_____

_____

Body #2: Again, pick the most powerful one and turn it into a succinct body paragraph:

_____

_____

_____

_____

_____

_____

_____

_____

_____

_____

_____

_____

Body #3: Brainstorm for your second trait:

_____

_____

_____

_____

_____

_____

Body #3: Pick the most powerful story and turn it into a succinct body paragraph:

_____

_____

_____

_____

_____

_____

_____

_____

_____

_____

_____

Body #4: Brainstorm stories for your third and final trait:

_____

_____

_____

_____

_____

_____

_____

Body #4: Once more, pick the most powerful one and turn it into a succinct body paragraph:

_____

_____

_____

_____

_____

_____

_____

_____

_____

_____

_____

Body Paragraphs Checklist:

- [ ] First body paragraph (answering the "why medicine" question) has a convincing anecdote in support of this.

  - [ ] You play an active role in this anecdote.

  - [ ] You zero in on details as much as possible in this anecdote.

- [ ] Second body paragraph (highlighting the first trait showcasing "why you will be an excellent physician") has a convincing anecdote in support of this.

  - [ ] You play an active role in this anecdote.

  - [ ] You zero in on details as much as possible in this anecdote.

- [ ] Third body paragraph (highlighting the second trait showcasing "why you will be an excellent physician") has a convincing anecdote in support of this.

  - [ ] You play an active role in this anecdote.

  - [ ] You zero in on details as much as possible in this anecdote.

- [ ] Fourth body paragraph (highlighting the third trait showcasing why you will be an excellent physician) has a convincing anecdote in support of this.

  - [ ] You play an active role in this anecdote.

  - [ ] You zero in on details as much as possible in this anecdote.

Up Next: Let's finish your introductory paragraph by adding a hook to your thesis that'll make sure we capture the reader's attention right out of the gate...

Step 3 – Finish Your Introductory Paragraph

Now that you have written the thesis to your introductory paragraph, all that remains is a hook. Intuitively enough, the hook is what captures the reader's attention which will ultimately help make your personal statement memorable. Remember: admissions committee members are reading thousands of essays, so how can you make your initial impression stand-out?

To start, we thought it would be pertinent to include examples of both good and bad introductory paragraphs. Of course, critiques will follow each example. Here is what NOT to do:

As a child, I always knew I wanted to be a doctor! If I saw a heart-tugging television ad about impoverished children, I wanted to help. I wanted to be making a difference in their lives. Therefore, for as long as I can remember, I have wanted to chase my dream of being a doctor to serve those around me.

This hook is simply too cliché. The hook should have personal relevance to you, and that will hopefully make it unique. Thousands upon thousands of applicants could write the same exact story above – and actually do. So, don't be like them! Now, let's take a look at a better example:

Growing up, I was the child with the never-ending "whys" that exasperated my parents. While I can answer why metoclopramide should not be prescribed to a Parkinson's patient, I do not know why particular symptoms and test results constitute a diagnosis or warrant certain treatment. I want to become a doctor because medicine is where I can answer these questions, ultimately venturing further. Given my thoroughness, teamwork skills, motivational skills, and the pharmacology knowledge I have fine-tuned over the past 10 years, the medical profession and I are a perfect fit.

This introductory paragraph from a current pharmacist interested in pursuing medicine uniquely hooks the reader. He skilfully relates the "whys" of his childhood to the current "whys" in his adult life. Then, a single sentence suffices to segue to his thesis. Notice how this thesis answers both the "why medicine" and the "why you will excel in the field" questions; while the previous attempt only answers the "why medicine" question.

Moving on, there are two ways to go about the global personal statement organization: either have an overarching theme for the entire personal statement, or simply a story in the introduction that entices the reader. Which you choose is a matter of writing style and preference.

An important element of the hook is to either create some emotion in the reader or an intense desire/curiosity to continue reading. To further illustrate, your first few sentences should give a slight, but savory taste that is just enough to leave them hungry for more.

That being said, brainstorm unique ways to hook your audience (that have personal relevance to you):

_____

_____

_____

_____

_____

_____

_____

Now, pick the most thrilling idea from above and turn it into the remainder of your introductory paragraph. The key is to be concise. You want to quickly hook your reader and then leave them with your thesis statement, which again, is your core argument for the personal statement. The meat of your paper lies in the body paragraphs, where you prove your thesis. Now, write your finished introductory paragraph:

_____

_____

_____

_____

_____

_____

_____

_____

_____

_____

Don't forget to add your thesis as the last sentence of your introductory paragraph

Introductory Paragraph Checklist:

☐ Your hook is not cliché.

☐ Your hook actually relates to your pursuit of medicine.

☐ Your hook captivates the reader.

☐ You segue quickly and smoothly to your thesis statement.

Up Next: Let's finish your essay on a high-note by creating a powerful concluding paragraph...

Step 4 – Write Your Concluding Paragraph

Congratulations! All the hard work is over and you have just one final step to complete your personal statement rough draft. It is safe to say that the concluding paragraph is by-far the most simple section to write. You are NOT introducing any new information. The scope of the paper has already been defined by the thesis and expanded upon by the body paragraphs. Instead, you are summarizing the ideas of your thesis and body paragraphs and then closing with a unique, rewritten version of your thesis. This leaves the argument – why you have chosen medicine and why you will be an amazing physician – fresh in your reader's mind. It sounds simple, but it's hard to mess this section up if you follow those simple rules.

Finish your personal statement by writing your concluding paragraph (remember to try to put a unique spin on your thesis without bringing in any new ideas):

_____

_____

_____

_____

_____

_____

_____

_____

_____

_____

_____

_____

Concluding Paragraph checklist

☐ No new information is introduced in the concluding paragraph.

☐ Previously mentioned ideas (from body paragraphs) are summarized briefly.

☐ You close with a reworked version of your thesis.

Up Next: Now that you have solid rough draft in the bag, it's time to polish-up your essay so that it's ready to make a strong impression and get you into medical school...

Step 5 – Above and Beyond: Turning A Good Essay Into A Great One

Trust me, to leverage the power of the personal statement, you don't just want to settle for a good essay, you want an amazing one! A good personal statement will merely reside among the thousands of other good personal statements. An amazing one will make the admissions member really want to dive further into your application and also make all the difference when they are on the fence regarding your acceptance. To help you and your essay achieve greatness, in this last step we'll:

- ✓ Outline the importance of feedback and how/where to get it.

- ✓ Review the final "dos and don'ts" regarding the medical school personal statement.

- ✓ Give you the opportunity to review your own essay by providing "Bryan's Black Bag's Rubric".

- ✓ Take you step-by-step through multiple drafts of a sample personal statement.

- ✓ Plus, we've added on two, fully annotated personal statements!

Importance of Quality Feedback

After making your way through this book, and completing the worksheets, you should have a respectable personal statement draft. That being said, I can promise you that there still is work to be done. Those that have the grit to write a myriad of drafts to perfect their essay are the ones that are most memorable and thus stand the best chance of getting accepted into medical school. Don't get discouraged though, it will all come together and ultimately be worth it!

Who should I have review my personal statement? (It's important to reiterate this FAQ addressed earlier)

"There are two types of edits: those grammatical in nature, which touch on punctuation and syntax, and those that zero in on content. In the case of the personal statement, that content is going to revolve around how well your body paragraphs support your thesis statement. The grammar edit can be done by anyone with a proficient English background. These are not the types of edits that will truly transform your personal statement though. It is your choice of content and the delivery of supporting stories (don't worry, there is much more on this to follow!) that really elevates a personal statement to something truly special. Therefore, the pool of people who can provide critical content insight is much more limited. An obvious starting point is other premeds, but you ideally want someone who has successfully matriculated, as that shows they understand what is necessary to create a strong personal statement. Some schools have pre-med advisers, but unfortunately not all are cut from the same cloth. I was truly blessed to have an incredible pre-med adviser who continually provided invaluable insight and feedback. This is not the case at all institutions and you will be left to determine for yourself whether your adviser can provide what you need. Last, there are reputable companies out there than can turn your personal statement from an average submission into one that is truly magnificent.

Honestly, receiving quality feedback from different points of view will make all the difference in the effectiveness of your final draft. So please don't forget this pivotal step!

Final Dos and Don'ts

Now that you are an expert on the personal statement, having a respectable first draft, you could probably construct a quality table of dos and don'ts. To save you time though, we have gone ahead and done that for you! Give this a quick glance and make sure you accomplished the dos and avoided the don'ts.

Dos	Don'ts
Write a persuasive, thesis-driven essay.	Write a narrative of your entire life, lacking a thesis.
Entice your audience with an engaging hook relevant to you.	Use a dramatic hook with no clear relation to you.
Answer the relevant questions in the thesis (why medicine and why you will be a kick-ass physician).	Fail to answer the relevant questions in your thesis, or lack a thesis.
Organize body paragraphs chronologically with respect to your thesis.	Organize body paragraphs haphazardly.
Use active anecdotes, zeroing in on details, for each body paragraph.	Leave anecdotes and details out of body paragraphs or fail to use active anecdotes, opting for passive ones instead.
Focus on 1-2 anecdotes per body paragraph, allowing for proper development of them.	List many undeveloped anecdotes in body paragraphs, making them read more like a resume than a persuasive essay.
Revisit the ideas already discussed in the concluding paragraph.	Introduce new information in the concluding paragraph.
Close with a fresh, rewritten version of your thesis.	Fail to close with a reworked thesis, which leaves your argument (why medicine and why you will be a kick-ass physician) unclear in the reader's mind.

Review Your Own Essay

If your essay doesn't live up to your own standards, what are the chances it will live up to an admissions committee? It's important to be honest with yourself when filling out this rubric, and critical for others to fill this out as well.

Introductory Paragraph

1) Does the hook (the first few sentences of the introductory paragraph) actually hook you?

      1   2   3   4   5   6   7   8   9   10

2) Is the hook concise and to the point?

      1   2   3   4   5   6   7   8   9   10

3) Does the hook segue smoothly into the thesis?

      1   2   3   4   5   6   7   8   9   10

4) Does the thesis answer why the writer is interested in medicine, as well as why they will be an excellent physician?

      1   2   3   4   5   6   7   8   9   10

Body Paragraph One

1) Does the topic sentence relate back to the thesis chronologically, meaning: is this the first idea mentioned chronologically in the thesis?

      1   2   3   4   5   6   7   8   9   10

2) Does the writer take an active role in the stories and/or insights mentioned in the body paragraph (are they the one the story centers on or are they the one arriving at the insights)?

      1   2   3   4   5   6   7   8   9   10

3) Do the stories and/or insights zero in on details as much as possible, rather than giving a broad overview?

      1   2   3   4   5   6   7   8   9   10

4) Are you convinced by the stories and/or insights of what the applicant is trying to prove in this paragraph?

1　　2　　3　　4　　5　　6　　7　　8　　9　　10

Body Paragraph Two

1) Does the topic sentence relate back to the thesis chronologically, meaning: is this the second idea mentioned chronologically in the thesis?

1　　2　　3　　4　　5　　6　　7　　8　　9　　10

2) Does the writer take an active role in the stories and/or insights mentioned in the body paragraph (are they the one the story centers on, and are they the one arriving at the insights)?

1　　2　　3　　4　　5　　6　　7　　8　　9　　10

3) Do the stories and/or insights zero in on details as much as possible, rather than giving a broad overview?

1　　2　　3　　4　　5　　6　　7　　8　　9　　10

4) Are you convinced by the stories and/or insights of what the applicant is trying to prove in this paragraph?

1　　2　　3　　4　　5　　6　　7　　8　　9　　10

Body Paragraph Three

1) Does the topic sentence relate back to the thesis chronologically, meaning: is this the third idea mentioned chronologically in the thesis?

1　　2　　3　　4　　5　　6　　7　　8　　9　　10

2) Does the writer take an active role in the stories and/or insights mentioned in the body paragraph (are they the one the story centers on, and are they the one arriving at the insights)?

1　　2　　3　　4　　5　　6　　7　　8　　9　　10

3) Do the stories and/or insights zero in on details as much as possible, rather than giving a broad overview?

1　　2　　3　　4　　5　　6　　7　　8　　9　　10

4) Are you convinced by the stories and/or insights of what the applicant is trying to prove in this paragraph?

1　　2　　3　　4　　5　　6　　7　　8　　9　　10

Body Paragraph Four

1) Does the topic sentence relate back to the thesis chronologically, meaning: is this the fourth idea mentioned chronologically in the thesis?

     1   2   3   4   5   6   7   8   9   10

2) Does the writer take an active role in the stories and/or insights mentioned in the body paragraph (are they the one the story centers on, and are they the one arriving at the insights)?

     1   2   3   4   5   6   7   8   9   10

3) Do the stories and/or insights zero in on details as much as possible, rather than giving a broad overview?

     1   2   3   4   5   6   7   8   9   10

4) Are you convinced by the stories and/or insights of what the applicant is trying to prove in this paragraph?

     1   2   3   4   5   6   7   8   9   10

Closing Paragraph

1) Does the closing paragraph rehash information already presented, rather than introducing new ideas?

     1   2   3   4   5   6   7   8   9   10

2) Does the writer's rewritten thesis leave you with a strong sense of their initial argument?

     1   2   3   4   5   6   7   8   9   10

Overall

3) Ultimately, are you convinced of what they set out to prove in their thesis?

     1   2   3   4   5   6   7   8   9   10

Multiple Draft Essay Example

Rather than talk you through these finer-points, many of which have already been discussed in depth, I think it would be more prudent to actually show you the progression of a client I worked with.

NOTE: The comments/edits made below do not include any generic proofreading edits like grammar and punctuation, those of which would be included in any review package purchased.

What follows is Alyssia's personal statement, the first, second, and third drafts, with my actual comments. She is a talented writer to begin with, but also skillfully incorporated my philosophies into an extremely effective and memorable personal statement…

Alyssia's First Draft

As I opened my Snapchat app, I was engrossed. There were flashes - flashes of MRI scans, ten-second clips explaining the definition of chondromalacia, patient-specific skeletal models made from the latest 3D printing technology. A few emails later, I am sitting in the office of the physician who was distributing this captivating content on the latest social media platform. The connection I developed with a local radiologist resembles my unconventional journey to becoming a physician.

The purpose of the introduction is to draw the reader in with a unique and concise hook. It does not have to be particularly spectacular, like curing cancer, but it should certainly be memorable. Remember, the admissions committee member reading your personal statement is literally reading thousands. Make yours stand out.

After your hook, you need to segue into your thesis. Organization is crucial because it clearly and concisely sets out your argument, as well as the rest of the paper to provide evidence for said argument. With this in mind, the thesis should answer two questions. First, why are you interested in medicine? Second, why will you excel in this field?

Let's apply this to your intro. The hook definitely draws the reader in and is novel. Well done! As for the thesis, or what I believe to be the thesis, it needs some elaborating. You do not answer either of those questions, which is crucial to the piece. I recommend a single introductory paragraph, which quickly draws the reader in and then lays out your argument in the form of a thesis. This gives you ample characters for your body paragraphs, which is where you prove your thesis. This is the meat of the personal statement and where you can really drive your points home!

This part of my story began years ago. In college, all aspects of my most-beloved experiences pointed me towards medical school. First, I was driven by learning and gaining new experiences. With my explorative nature, I learned to grow cell lines in cancer research, monitored cardiovascular health in clinical studies, and analyzed patient DNA in a genetics laboratory. Second, I have greatly enjoyed making direct impacts and serving others through volunteering. I drafted sponsorship request letters for Ronald McDonald House Charities, utilized an online system to order groceries for elderly in need, chatted with patients and their loved ones in the hospital, and rocked children to sleep in the local homeless shelter. Because the changing field of medicine and complexity of patient care requires that primary care providers have an inquisitive outlook, open mind, fresh perspectives, and strong desire to the improve the community, I believed I had found my niche and applied to medical school during my last undergraduate year.

As I noted above, the body paragraphs follow the organizational scheme set forth in your thesis statement. You answer two questions, why are you interested in medicine and why will you do great things in this field? The evidence that you lay out in your thesis becomes the body paragraphs, as you expound upon it there. I would recommend a maximum of four body paragraphs to be able to fully develop each idea.

Again, your thesis is under-developed, which translates to subsequent body paragraphs being under-developed. You need to introduce why you are interested in medicine first. Then, this body paragraph will expand upon that. Second, this body paragraph merely reads like a list. That is not the point of a personal statement. You should pick two (or a maximum of three) ideas supporting why you want to be a physician. Then, support each one with some concrete evidence. You mention all the things you have done that have fueled your passion for medicine, but you do not dive into the details. Diving into the details is what I refer to as showing, rather than telling the reader. This is how you write a powerful personal statement. So, make this read like a personal statement body paragraph, rather than an uninspiring list.

Over the last two years, I have spent a great deal of time reflecting on my commitment to the profession and expanding my level of experience to become a more prepared and competitive applicant. I have been working as a clinical laboratory technologist, and while I thoroughly enjoy the team-based environment, my interest has remained on human connection. With hopes of gaining more direct patient-care experience, I trained in phlebotomy in my spare time last year. It felt fulfilling exiting each patient room. Working closely with skilled phlebotomists, we were part of the healthcare team, interacting with nurses and the lab. We were friends, listening intently to small talk and memories with patients. We were focused, aiming to yield successful draws that would result in the least discomfort, the most accurate results, and best serve the patients. It was a great challenge, but fulfilling to discover the importance of our short-lived, but long-impacting connections and relationships with patients. As a result, I knew I wanted to expand my role in the healthcare team.

This is precisely what I mean by showing, rather than telling. You get into the guts of your experience as a phlebotomist, highlighting your compassionate nature. This is how the previous paragraph needs to be crafted. Moreover, you should really only dedicate one body paragraph to your interest in medicine. The remaining body paragraphs should be devoted to the second vital question answered by the thesis: why will you be an outstanding physician? You could still use this experience but highlight how your compassionate nature will allow you to succeed as a physician.

Observing a variety of physicians, my connection to this position grew stronger, and during each observation, I was struck by the knowledgeable, team-oriented providers I hoped to emulate. Their ability to inform, reassure, listen, and discuss with patients strengthened my aspiration to pursue this career. Hoping to spend more time observing patient-provider interactions and gain a deeper understanding of the profession, I began scribing for an orthopedic surgeon. Again, I had the opportunity to listen to more patient stories, this time in a different capacity. During follow-up visits, the long-term connections made were ones I hoped to emulate. In booking surgeries, the thorough analysis was a challenge I hoped to take on. As individuals smiled after joint replacements, I wished to bring such joy into the lives of others.

The problem here is that you highlight little to nothing about yourself. You are the applicant, not the physician you work for. It is totally fine to highlight things you observed him or her do that were worth emulating, but then you need to show how you put them into practice. Again, this requires showing the reader through a concrete example.

My commitment to becoming a physician stems from the gratification of working with patients and the community; however, my devotion remains due to the distinctions of the position. Physicians are leaders, yet they retain the support of the healthcare team. As a laboratory technologist, there is satisfaction in complex decision-making and working independently, but I appreciate the team-based collaborative environment. Primary care providers also have the priceless opportunity of lifelong learning. Having been fortunate to have had such a wide variety of experiences in volunteering, research, clinical sciences, and healthcare, I deeply value any opportunity to expand my understanding and knowledge base. With innovative techniques, updated technology, and improving procedures there is always more to learn in the field of medicine, which intrigues me and fuels my desire to learn. Most importantly, physicians put the needs of the patient first as a holistic patient-care provider. Advocating for better laboratory practices to improve efficiency of providing patient results, maintaining specificity and thoughtful consideration during each patient visit to create accurate visit notes while scribing, and taking the time to provide comfort to patients before a difficult draw as a phlebotomist are each experiences that have prepared me to take on this responsibility.

Again, there is way too much going on in one body paragraph. You have multiple ideas: physicians as leaders, lifelong learning, and putting the needs of the patient first. The body paragraphs need to have more narrow focuses. This is what allows you to fully develop each idea. Right now, you simply do not have the space to develop these ideas with concrete anecdotes. As a result, I am left unconvinced. Additionally, you are still yet to talk about why you will be a good physician. The entire piece is about your interest in medicine, which is only half of the equation.

I look forward to expanding my role in the stories of others by becoming a physician. It has been a gratifying experience to work in many different aspects of healthcare over the years. Everything from laboratory research, to hospital volunteering, and now to scribing has been educational, challenging, and most of all, satisfying. In a profession of endless possibilities with incredible opportunities, I am confident that my experiences and dedication have prepared me for the lifelong journey of a physician.

The concluding paragraph should be the simplest paragraph to write in your personal statement. This is not a place for new information; instead, you are merely revisiting things that you have discussed previously (the evidence that you expanded upon in your body paragraphs) and then closing with a rewritten version of your thesis to remind the reader of your argument: why you are interested in medicine and why you will be a fantastic physician.

With respect to this, you follow this recipe. The remainder of the piece needs some work though, so I would loop back around to the conclusion when that is in order.

The personal statement is a tough beast to tackle. I wrote several drafts myself, eventually losing count. Don't dismay, just keep working at it! Here are my recommendations for proceeding with the second draft:

1. You need to develop a thesis statement. This encompasses your argument for the piece. First, why you are interested in medicine and second, why you will do fantastic things in this field. Reflect on the evidence you wish to use to support this argument, as it will lay the groundwork for the body paragraphs to follow. In this manner, the thesis is truly the road map to the entire piece, with your body paragraphs following suit.

2. As governed by the thesis, each body paragraph needs to have a specific focus. You are simply expanding on the evidence put forth in your thesis. The most powerful way to do this is to show the reader, not tell them why you possess X, Y, or Z. Zeroing in on a particular anecdote or story is how we recommend doing this. This draws the reader in and convinces them beyond a shadow of a doubt. On the other hand, if you do not have an anecdote or story, or it is poorly developed, then the reader is left unconvinced. One more piece of advice is to employ active examples for this. By active examples, I mean that you are the one the story focuses on, rather than you passively observing someone else being great or doing fantastic things. Remember, you are the applicant!

3. Last, the concluding paragraph will simply tie the evidence in your body paragraphs back together. Then, it closes with a fresh version of your thesis, leaving the reader with your argument once more (why medicine and why you will make a great doctor).

Alyssia's Second Draft

As I opened my Snapchat app, I was hooked. There were short flashes - flashes of MRI scans, ten second clips explaining the definition of chondromalacia, and patient-specific skeletal models made from the latest 3D printing technology. Emails later, I am sitting in the office of the physician who was distributing this captivating content on the latest social media platform, ready to shadow his work in person. Developing this unconventional contact with a local radiologist represents my dedicated pursuit of knowledge, fresh perspective, and desire to make meaningful connections as I pursue medicine with the hopes of leading improvements in my community and investigating complex cases as a physician.

This is a beauty. You have a concise, certainly unique hook that relates to your journey into medicine. Then, you answer why you want to be a doctor: to make improvements in your community and investigate complex cases. Moreover, you also answer why you will be a good physician: your dedicated pursuit of knowledge, fresh perspective, and desire to make meaningful connections.

Through the years, my most beloved experiences have included working in different capacities with my community. Growing up, I was a fixture in family businesses providing services in our motels and coffee shops. Entering college, this translated to an interest in volunteering. I met Donna at the Ronald McDonald House and looked forward to working on our to-do list in the office each week. I remember Sammy, laughing over a game of Candyland while she visits her mother in the hospital. Richard ordered a cream cake every time we chatted during his grocery order. Thinking fondly of these individuals, it is connections like these that inspire me to work with my community in a greater capacity as a physician.

You are on the right track here. This body paragraph parallels your thesis, wanting to become a physician to positively impact your community. Rather than haphazardly throwing in all these people you volunteered with though, stick to a max of two and make the paragraph a bit longer to develop these relationships. For instance, who is Donna? A patient at the Ronald McDonald House? Also, who is Sammy? They certainly deserve more than one sentence. Give the reader something to sink their teeth into.

Physicians are allowed this priceless opportunity to work with the community on a regular basis, but the position also consists of the puzzling challenges that entice me. The day I got the email that I could volunteer for a summer in cancer research, I remember I could not contain my smile. The weeks of organizing data, constructing my plans for testing, and analyzing my work were long, but fulfilling. Though the research ended without conclusive evidence, the thought of that experience still excites me. It was my own puzzle to solve by devising my own structured course in the most efficient way I could create. With the complex science in healthcare and patients having the most variable set of contained factors, medicine is a challenge I would be excited to take on every day.

No critiques here. Again, this parallels your thesis. Moreover, you have a solid example supporting your claim that you aspire to be a doctor in part because of the unique challenge it poses. Well done!

Since graduating college, I have aimed to prepare myself for taking on the dense field of medicine. Working as a clinical laboratory technologist has developed my ability to work in a complex team-based setting. On busy nights, it can be a balancing act maintaining efficiency of independent testing while consulting others on quantifying a questionable result. We promote organization, adaptability, and constant communication in training new techs because this is the core of our success as a cohesive unit. The team has given me the opportunity to lead in generating positive group discussion, advocate for better laboratory practices to improve efficiency for our patients and take on challenges in collaboration in a clinical setting.

You do a solid job of demonstrating your ability to work in a cohesive environment. Your thesis outlines your dedicated pursuit of knowledge next though. Remember, this is the road map to the entire piece; thus, you should change the thesis to reflect what you actually talk about here. This is a simple fix though!

Working closely with others has shown me the importance of taking on new perspectives, a mindset I utilized in taking on a part-time role as a Medical Scribe. As I observed each visit, I learned the ways in which the provider conducted patient interviews and physical exams. Understanding what the provider was looking for with each question and each touch, I developed my own system in formulating effective visit notes. Equipping myself with the required knowledge and skills to compose patient stories but knowing there is always more to learn and improve upon, is an aspect of medicine that I find alluring. Continuing to challenge myself with new experiences and stepping outside of my comfort zone, I am confidently prepared to take on the medical field.

Again, this is well written and conveys your adaptability! This is picky, but your thesis outlines fresh perspective as the next body paragraph. I am not sure this descriptor appropriately describes what you are talking about here. Perhaps something more along the lines of expanding your perspective by continually broadening your horizons would be nice.

Aside from working to improve patient stories from the laboratory, documenting them as a scribe, and listening to them as a volunteer/shadow, I played a role within the stories as a phlebotomy student. Most memorably, while in the hospital, there was an elderly gentleman we had to stick. He had been poked earlier that day, and you could see the markings on his skin from previous draws. He was talking with the physical therapist as I moved about the room preparing and trying not to disrupt his attention. It was obvious he was not keen on having his blood drawn again, and it was difficult to find a good location. My trainer nodded as I reached for a heat pack and placed it over his hand. The goal was a successful draw with minimal discomfort, and careful preparation paid off as the collection was done without a sound from the patient. As I wrapped him, he looked over briefly and gave a short smile before returning to his conversation. In those few moments, I felt I had accomplished a great deal and that overwhelming sense of fulfillment gives me the confidence to continue in my pursuit of medicine. Always known as the hard worker, my experiences in healthcare have given me undying drive to push to work harder.

You say you felt as if you had accomplished a great deal and you certainly had. Put a name to it though! What did you accomplish? This will make it easier for the readier to grasp onto and clearly relate this anecdote back to the thesis. With respect to the last sentence, don't close with hard-work. This paragraph is about your desire for meaningful connections!

I look forward to expanding my role in the stories of others by becoming a physician. It has been a gratifying experience to work in many different aspects of healthcare over the years. Everything from laboratory research, to hospital volunteering, and now to scribing has been educational, challenging, and most of all, satisfying. In a profession of endless possibilities with incredible opportunities, I am confident that my experiences and dedication have prepared me for the lifelong journey of a physician.

I can honestly say this is one of the best personal statements I have read. You really took my previous advice to heart and the result is absolutely beautiful! With the minor tweaks I have outlined, this bad boy is ready for submission!

Alyssia's Final Draft

As I opened my Snapchat app, I was hooked. There were flashes - flashes of MRI scans, ten second clips explaining the definition of chondromalacia, and patient-specific skeletal models made from the latest 3D printing technology. Emails later, I am sitting in the office of the physician who was distributing this captivating content on the latest social media platform ready to shadow his work in person. Developing this unconventional contact with a local radiologist represents my ability to adapt in expanding my perspective, my openness to challenging myself with new experiences, and my desire to make meaningful connections. I pursue medicine with the hopes of leading improvements in my community and investigating complex cases as a physician.

Through the years, my most beloved experiences have included working in different capacities with my community. Growing up, I was a fixture in family businesses providing services in our motels and coffee shops. In college, this translated to an interest in volunteering. I met Donna, Director of Sponsorships, at the Ronald McDonald House and looked forward to working on our to-do list each week. I expected to learn about Microsoft and bookkeeping, but found myself simply enjoying her company. I also remember Sam, a young girl, sitting alone in the waiting room as I volunteered in a local hospital. She was visiting her mother who was recovering from surgery, and we bonded over a love of board games, laughing over countless rounds of Candyland. Thinking fondly of these individuals, it is connections like these that inspire me to work with my community in a greater capacity as a physician.

Physicians are allowed this priceless opportunity to work with the community on a regular basis, but the position also consists of puzzling challenges that entice me. The day I got the email that I could volunteer for a summer in cancer research, I remember I could not contain my smile. The weeks of organizing data, constructing my plans for testing, and analyzing my work were long, but fulfilling. Though the research ended without conclusive evidence, the thought of that experience still excites me. It was my own puzzle to solve by devising my own structured course in the most efficient way I could create. With the complex science in healthcare and patients having the most variable set of contained factors, medicine is a challenge I would be excited to take on every day.

Since graduating college, I have aimed to prepare myself for tackling the dense field of medicine. Working as a clinical lab technologist has developed my ability to work in a complex team-based setting. On busy nights, it can be a balancing act, maintaining efficiency of independent testing while consulting others on quantifying a questionable result. We promote organization, adaptability, and constant communication in training new techs because this is the core of our success as a cohesive unit. The team has given me the opportunity to lead in generating positive group discussion, advocate for better lab practices to improve efficiency for our patients, and take on challenges in collaboration in a clinical setting.

Working closely with others has shown me the importance of taking on new perspectives, a mindset I utilized in taking on a part-time role as a Medical Scribe. As I observed each visit, I learned the ways in which the provider conducted patient interviews and physical exams. Understanding what the provider was looking for with each question and touch, I developed my own system in formulating effective visit notes. Equipping myself with the required knowledge and skills to compose patient stories, but knowing there is always more to learn and improve upon, is an aspect of medicine I find alluring. Continuing to challenge myself with new experiences and stepping outside of my comfort zone, I am confidently prepared to take on the medical field.

Aside from working to improve patient stories from the lab, documenting them as a scribe, and listening to them as a volunteer, I played a role within the stories as a phlebotomy student. Most memorably, while in the hospital, there was an elderly gentleman we had to stick. I could see the markings on his skin from previous draws as I prepared. It was obvious he was not keen on having his blood drawn again, and it was difficult to find a good location. My trainer nodded as I reached for a heat pack and placed it over his hand. The goal was a successful draw with minimal discomfort, and careful preparation paid off as the collection was done without a sound from the patient. As I wrapped him, he looked over briefly and gave a smile before returning to his conversation. In those few moments, I felt I had accomplished a great deal in providing care with the utmost respect for comfort.

I look forward to expanding my role in the stories of others by becoming a physician. It has been a gratifying experience to work in many aspects of healthcare over the years. Everything from lab research, to hospital volunteering, and now scribing has been educational, challenging, and most of all satisfying. In a profession of endless possibilities, I am confident that my experiences and dedication have prepared me for the lifelong journey of a physician.

Closing Remarks

I am extremely grateful you decided to purchase this workbook and hope that you were satisfied with the quality you received. I was once a pre-med in your position and can relate to how daunting and uncertain this whole process may seem. And unfortunately, many applicants that are truly passionate about medicine get discouraged and start to lose confidence in themselves and their hope of becoming a doctor. I've got your back and am here whenever you need me! Let's have the next generation of doctors be the best generation of doctors!

Have any feedback for me? I would love for any reviews/feedback on how to make this book better for future pre-meds. Your feedback will make a huge difference, so I want to thank you in advance! I can be reached at my personal email address (bryanmiles17@gmail.com), twitter account (@Bryans_BlackBag), or medical school blog (bryansblackbag.com). Additionally, I have a YouTube channel (Bryan's Black Bag) full of advice for premeds, med students, and beyond!

Extras: Example Personal Statement One

I have included my own personal statement to demonstrate all the above principles. My personal statement is by no means perfect, but I wrote it with these guidelines in mind, so hopefully it will be of some use to you. I have commentary after each paragraph. Enjoy:

I vividly remember driving up the entrance to Gustavus Adolphus College. It was freshmen year and upperclassmen, appropriately coined "Gustie Greeters," vibrantly welcomed my family and I to campus. Starting college was an unnerving yet welcomed adventure. Little did I know this special community would engrain three core values, full effort, positive attitude, and empathy, all the while revealing the intimacy between medicine and the human condition. My mission was clear then and continues to be reaffirmed as a scribe at Twin Cities Orthopedics (TCO). I want to become a physician because it is a unique way of serving people, as well as sharing my three guiding life philosophies.

I begin with the hook, describing my welcoming experience at Gustavus Adolphus. I choose this hook because this was a special community that truly shaped me as a person, engraining the three core values I mentioned. Organization is crucial in a personal statement. That is why I introduce my three core values here, as well as my experience at Twin Cities Orthopedics, all of which become standalone body paragraphs. Moreover, I touch on how these core values illuminated the unique nature of medicine. This serves as a prelude to my thesis, which answers the two vital questions. First, why do I want to be a doctor? Because it is a unique way of serving people. Second, why will I thrive in this field? Because I will share my three guiding life philosophies.

The Gustavus tennis coaches helped instill my first core value, full effort. They demanded focus every second, which translated to the unparalleled opportunity for improvement. Our team adopted this philosophy, pushing each other toward our greatest potential. This was best exemplified by fitness, which we viewed as a healthy intra-team competition. I brought this attitude into all aspects of my life. As a chemistry tutor, full effort was essential. My students had a variety of needs, but one stands out. She struggled most with the laboratory component. One night, we spent three hours combing over a complex experiment. She left our session not only comprehending the lab, but also with a renewed vigor to tackle next week's experiment. In short, full effort entails inspiration of others. This is certainly appropriate within medicine, where patients are in trying situations. As a physician, I will inspire my patients to their greatest potential through full effort.

The thesis is truly the road map for the personal statement. That is why the ideas introduced there become the body paragraphs. My first core value was full effort; therefore, this paragraph is about full effort. I discuss where it was fine-tuned, the tennis court, and then delve into an example of utilizing it elsewhere. I say "show, don't tell" in my critiques. Here is what I mean by that. I "show" my full effort in describing the hours I spent with my student as well as the positive impact this had on her. It is much more powerful than merely saying I am a hard worker. Last, I relate full effort back to medicine, discussing how I will inspire future patients. This is something that is often left out with closing sentences to body paragraphs. Don't forget to bring everything full circle!

Positive attitude, my second core value, was best exemplified by Steve Wilkinson, one of my tennis coaches who recently succumbed to metastatic cancer. From the onset of his terminal diagnosis, he sported an ear-to-ear grin and palpable optimism. Only minutes in his presence would lift anyone's spirits. Living far beyond his six-month prognosis, he is a reminder of the power of medicine in preserving life, but also the devastation of disease. Steve was never unrealistic about his health, but eternal positivity allowed him to live in the moment for his final years. Inspired by Steve, I have used this mindset countless times. On one occasion, friends rushed my girlfriend to the local ER due to her life-threatening food allergy. I quickly followed. Nora was almost unrecognizable, covered from head to toe in red, blotchy hives. She was in panic and, given her already labored breathing, I knew I had to try to calm her down. I grabbed her puffy hand and watched her slowly relax as I reiterated that she was in very capable hands. Experiencing medicine from this perspective has taught me to never underestimate the power of positivity. I am excited to be a beacon of positive energy within the lives of my future patients.

As you can see, the second element of my thesis, positive attitude, becomes the second paragraph. Another critique we often mention when reviewing personal statements is to utilize active examples, not passive ones. An active example highlights a story where you and your actions are the focal point or showcases your strengths. Passive examples show you watching someone else being great. They are not as powerful in making you stand out as an applicant. Passive examples can certainly be woven into your statement, as long as they are followed by an active example showing that you internalized the trait. That is what I did here. I talk about learning the power of positivity from my coach and then how I embodied this when my girlfriend (now wife ☺) wound up in the emergency room. Again, I close the paragraph by relating this to medicine and how I will embody this for future patients as well.

Empathy, my final core value, was built upon by Dr. Koepke, an ER physician I shadowed for several years. An ER is the first line of defense against trauma and illness. Well aware of this, Dr. Koepke proceeded with boundless compassion when one gentleman fell off a ladder and severely dislocated his shoulder. Despite pain medication, he was in agony. Dr. Koepke caringly and reassuringly grasped his good shoulder, telling him everything was going to be okay. Ease washed over the patient's face and relocation alleviated much of his pain. Working in the memory care unit of a local nursing home as a CNA, empathy was essential. Each shift, I was responsible for up to ten residents. I devotedly mastered their care plans, embedded with idiosyncrasies. I knew that Carol preferred a different lotion brand on certain body parts, while Evelyn desired her stuffed animal to receive grooming before herself. Incorporating these details, I darted from resident to resident for the duration of my shift. As a physician, I will care for my future patients in this manner.

You have no doubt glimpsed the pattern here. This third paragraph is devoted to my third core value, the third idea set forth in my thesis. As I did in the second paragraph, I lead with a passive example, viewing Dr. Koepke's empathy first-hand, then switching gears to an active example focused on me.

Working for physicians as a scribe at TCO has given me further insight into the profession. For instance, the full effort of physicians encompasses their role as educators. Working with Dr. Riggi, a Gustavus graduate himself, I have observed him meticulously explaining diagnoses with models, staying in the room until he is sure patients and family understand. Furthermore, I have seen how a physician's positive attitude can have a tremendous impact on a patient's recovery. Dr. Johnson, another physician I work with, certainly realizes this and inspires his patients to their full potential. Finally, trusting doctor-patient relationships begin with compassion. Since the physicians are immediately privy to intimate details, perhaps not even knowing the patient, empathy is vital to earning trust. Numerous TCO physicians I work for internalize this, building rewarding dynamics with their patients. I aspire to deliver the same standard of care.

The final idea in my thesis was how working at Twin Cities Orthopedics reaffirmed my desire to pursue medicine. Therefore, it became my fourth paragraph. Unfortunately, working as a scribe did not offer the opportunity for much direct patient care, thus I did not have any active examples to fall back on. Nonetheless, I thought it was very powerful that I saw my own core values being practiced by physicians on a daily basis. Therefore, I thought it was fitting to close with this body paragraph.

My experiences continue to cement my desire to become a physician. I know medicine is my calling because of its vigor in treating physical ailments, but also its special role as a medium for emotional care, namely through my core values: full effort, positive attitude, and empathy. As a provider, my care will center around these, one patient at a time.

The concluding paragraph should be the easiest to write. You do not need to introduce any new ideas, simply touch on everything that has been put forth already. I loop back around to my core values, restating my thesis with the second sentence.

Extras: Example Personal Statement Two

"This is it," I thought as I stared blankly at the freckles on my knees. I lay crouched against my parents' parked car on an unfamiliar street in Coronado, California. I swallowed hard as the painful swelling in my throat and tongue began to overwhelm my entire airway. "Relax, deep breaths," I repeated to myself as I firmly pressed an EpiPen into my thigh for the second time that afternoon. I was seventeen years old on a family vacation. I had begged my mother to allow me to eat a "vegan" chocolate cake – which, unfortunately, was not vegan enough; sending me into the worst anaphylactic shock I had ever experienced. Luckily, medicine prevailed.

Unlike my own personal statement introduction, which was a bit blander, this one really captivates the reader. It is important to note that you do not have to begin your personal statement with a medically enthralling anecdote. If you choose to go this route though, make sure it is something relevant and pertinent to your application. Obviously, this anecdote is highly personal, delving into a very traumatic life-threatening experience. If the relevance to you as an applicant is not apparent to the reader, then the introduction will fall short, no matter how well written.

Growing up with life-threatening food allergies has provided me with a unique exposure to medicine. This personal experience, combined with opportunities to conduct research, shadow physicians, volunteer, and participate in collegiate athletics has given me important insight into the intimate connection medicine forms between scientific endeavors and humanity.

This second introductory paragraph clearly states the relevance of the anecdote that drew the reader in. Nora's experience with life-threatening food allergies gave her unique insight into medicine. Then, she rounds out the thesis with various opportunities, including research, shadowing, volunteering, and collegiate athletics that have furthered her insight into medicine, specifically its intimacy with science and humanity. Ultimately, this is a nice example of a solid two-sentence thesis statement. The reader now has an idea of what is to follow, as the argument has been clearly laid out here.

"What can this possibly have to do with medicine?" I found myself wondering as I scribbled down reactions in my high school chemistry class. Thus far, my experience with health care consisted purely of the humanistic side; I could not understand how these seemingly cold, scientific facts fit into the equation. Consequently, when I was asked to lead a chemical research project in college, I was initially skeptical; however, my fondness for chemistry and respect for my mentor, Dr. Gardner, triumphed, and I accepted. The aim of the project was to synthesize a polymer with the potential for uses in medicine and nanotechnology. Dr. Gardner and I spent long hours and weekends trying and trying again, until finally, we had a breakthrough. We had synthesized a vital intermediate with an incredible, and yet-to-be reported, yield. I realized that many important

medical breakthroughs, like the Epipen, started in the lab. I could now understand what I failed to see in high school: the bigger picture. I am passionate about research because I realize that science has humanistic implications that are much larger than simply cold, hard, scientific facts.

Stemming from the thesis, we know this first body paragraph will be about research, moreover its link to medicine. She begins flashing back to high school. I always mention that high school experiences are irrelevant, but they are totally appropriate if utilized to lay groundwork for future experiences, as done here. When she discusses her basic science research, it is important to note how she does not delve into the nuts and bolts. That is not the point of this body paragraph and will likely be lost on most readers. Instead, she highlights the big picture application, which anybody reading this can sink their teeth into. Finally, bringing this paragraph full circle, since the point is to connect research to monumental medical breakthroughs, she mentions how the EpiPen (which saved her life) started similarly in a basic science laboratory.

I also discovered, through extensive time shadowing physicians, that it is the human interactions that separate clinics from laboratories. I had the experience of observing open heart surgery at the Aspirus Wausau Hospital. My own heart skipped a beat as I stood next to Dr. Miles while he repaired a man's mitral valve. The procedure was breathtaking. Equally striking was what I observed in the office. Dr. Miles' ability to explain procedures without complex medical jargon, commitment to never letting his patients feel rushed, and overall compassionate demeanor undoubtedly contributed to the adoration I saw from his patients. It was evident that he treats people as just that: people, not maladies to fix.

Now it is time to discuss shadowing. This paragraph is a passive experience, as all shadowing is. This is fine though, since the active internalization of it follows in the subsequent paragraph. Also, the insights she mentions, explaining procedures without convoluted medical jargon, never letting patients feel rushed during visits, and overall compassion, were actively arrived at. Therefore, when discussing passive examples, it is imperative that you highlight what you learned, somewhat rendering it an active experience. In this case, it is the unrivalled bedside manner of Dr. Miles.

After shadowing, I decided to take a more active role in medicine. I became a volunteer in the Emergency Department at the Mayo Clinic Health System-Mankato. My main duty is to improve the patient experience. One of my most memorable experiences occurred on my usual Sunday night shift from eight to midnight. I entered seven-year-old Emily's room to see if I could be of any assistance. Tears were streaming down her face as the doctor examined her wounded foot. She had stepped on a large amount of glass, and having it removed was going to be painful. I slipped out of her room and when I returned, pulled a teddy bear out from behind my back. "This teddy bear is only for very brave patients," I told her. "So you, Ms. Emily," I insisted, "must be very brave." She looked down at the teddy bear and beamed, her foot forgotten. My experience at Mayo has taught me that, in medicine, sometimes having all of the answers does not solve all of the problems. Often, people also need the comfort of another person.

And now we have the active internalization of what Nora witnessed while spending time with Dr. Miles. You can see here how she delves into a particular story that highlights the difference she made while volunteering. This is the most powerful way to convince the reader of your impact.

From Coronado, California, to a front-row seat in the OR, I have continually been inspired by the commitment, dedication, and teamwork I have witnessed in medicine. As a three-sport varsity athlete at Gustavus, these invaluable notions have become quite familiar to me. I learned commitment by continually pounding the pavement day after day in cross-country. I learned dedication by pushing past the pain in every 800-meter race I ran in track. I learned the necessity of teamwork through my 16 years of playing soccer. Athletics have enabled me to live a healthy lifestyle, develop communication skills, and learn the discipline that I believe will be vital in my future career.

Next in line are her collegiate athletics. The values she highlights – commitment, dedication, and teamwork – are all linked to respective sports. Moreover, she has an example, such as pounding the pavement in cross country. This evokes imagery and further convinces the reader, as opposed to simply saying commitment was ingrained through cross country.

My initial exposure to medicine through my allergies has given me a deep appreciation for physicians. As I lay on that unfamiliar street in Coronado, California, I thought that I might die, but thanks to medical assistance I did not. It turned out to be a pivotal event for me, giving rise to my passion for pursuing a career as a physician. My subsequent experiences conducting research, shadowing, volunteering and competing in varsity collegiate athletics have shown me the importance of compassion, teamwork and dedication. It is my highest aspiration to utilize these attributes to improve peoples' lives as a physician, while giving back to the community that has given me so much.

Now we come full circle. An option is to return to the anecdote mentioned initially, as the writer does here. Then she reiterates everything that has been discussed in the body paragraphs, including research, shadowing, volunteering, and collegiate athletics. Finally, she closes on a very heart-warming note, wanting to give back to the medical community that truly saved her life.

Extras: Grading Rubric

Introductory Paragraph

1) Does the hook (the first few sentences of the introductory paragraph) actually hook you?

    1   2   3   4   5   6   7   8   9   10

2) Is the hook concise and to the point?

    1   2   3   4   5   6   7   8   9   10

3) Does the hook segue smoothly into the thesis?

    1   2   3   4   5   6   7   8   9   10

4) Does the thesis answer why the writer is interested in medicine, as well as why they will be an excellent physician?

    1   2   3   4   5   6   7   8   9   10

Body Paragraph One

1) Does the topic sentence relate back to the thesis chronologically, meaning: is this the first idea mentioned chronologically in the thesis?

    1   2   3   4   5   6   7   8   9   10

2) Does the writer take an active role in the stories and/or insights mentioned in the body paragraph (are they the one the story centers on or are they the one arriving at the insights)?

    1   2   3   4   5   6   7   8   9   10

3) Do the stories and/or insights zero in on details as much as possible, rather than giving a broad overview?

    1   2   3   4   5   6   7   8   9   10

4) Are you convinced by the stories and/or insights of what the applicant is trying to prove in this paragraph?

1   2   3   4   5   6   7   8   9   10

Body Paragraph Two

1) Does the topic sentence relate back to the thesis chronologically, meaning: is this the second idea mentioned chronologically in the thesis?

1   2   3   4   5   6   7   8   9   10

2) Does the writer take an active role in the stories and/or insights mentioned in the body paragraph (are they the one the story centers on, and are they the one arriving at the insights)?

1   2   3   4   5   6   7   8   9   10

3) Do the stories and/or insights zero in on details as much as possible, rather than giving a broad overview?

1   2   3   4   5   6   7   8   9   10

4) Are you convinced by the stories and/or insights of what the applicant is trying to prove in this paragraph?

1   2   3   4   5   6   7   8   9   10

Body Paragraph Three

1) Does the topic sentence relate back to the thesis chronologically, meaning: is this the third idea mentioned chronologically in the thesis?

1   2   3   4   5   6   7   8   9   10

2) Does the writer take an active role in the stories and/or insights mentioned in the body paragraph (are they the one the story centers on, and are they the one arriving at the insights)?

1   2   3   4   5   6   7   8   9   10

3) Do the stories and/or insights zero in on details as much as possible, rather than giving a broad overview?

1   2   3   4   5   6   7   8   9   10

4) Are you convinced by the stories and/or insights of what the applicant is trying to prove in this paragraph?

1   2   3   4   5   6   7   8   9   10

Body Paragraph Four

1) Does the topic sentence relate back to the thesis chronologically, meaning: is this the fourth idea mentioned chronologically in the thesis?

1   2   3   4   5   6   7   8   9   10

2) Does the writer take an active role in the stories and/or insights mentioned in the body paragraph (are they the one the story centers on, and are they the one arriving at the insights)?

1   2   3   4   5   6   7   8   9   10

3) Do the stories and/or insights zero in on details as much as possible, rather than giving a broad overview?

1   2   3   4   5   6   7   8   9   10

4) Are you convinced by the stories and/or insights of what the applicant is trying to prove in this paragraph?

1   2   3   4   5   6   7   8   9   10

Closing Paragraph

1) Does the closing paragraph rehash information already presented, rather than introducing new ideas?

1   2   3   4   5   6   7   8   9   10

2) Does the writer's rewritten thesis leave you with a strong sense of their initial argument?

1   2   3   4   5   6   7   8   9   10

Overall

3) Ultimately, are you convinced of what they set out to prove in their thesis?

1   2   3   4   5   6   7   8   9   10